Fasting Your Way to Health

The Easy Way to Lose Weight & Live Longer

by Liz Armond

Published in UK by:

Liz Armond

© Copyright 2014 – Liz Armond

ISBN-13: 978-1512092172
ISBN-10: 1512092177

ALL RIGHTS RESERVED. No part of this publication may be reproduced or transmitted in any form whatsoever, electronic, or mechanical, including photocopying, recording, or by any informational storage or retrieval system without express written, dated and signed permission from the author.

Table of Contents

Introduction 1
Is Fasting a Good Idea? 3
How Our Body Works 5
What Makes a Lifestyle Unhealthy? 7
Fasting, What You Should Know 11
Other Uses and Facts About Fasting 15
    Medical application. 15
    Political application. 16
    Fast Facts About Fasting 17

Who Should NOT Fast? 19
Fasting for Health 21
Preparing to Fast 25
    Stages of Fasting 28

Additional Fasting Tips 31
Methods of Healthy Fasting 34
    Fasts that include foods 35
        Milk-Banana Diet 35
        Fruit Diet 36
        Fruit and Vegetable Diet 36
        Traditional Fast 36
    Fasts that do not include food 37
        Water Fast 37
        Complete Fast 38
        Juice fast 38

How to Fast Healthily? 41
Simple Fasting Program for Beginners 43
Easy Fasting & Detox Programs 49
    One Day Diet 49

    The Weekend Detox Diet 52
    7- Day Detox Diet 55

The 5:2 Fast Diet 63
    Lunch Menus 68
    Dinner Menus 71
    Additional Meals 77

Best Juicers 78
Conclusion 80
About the Author 82
Other Books by Author 83
Disclaimer and/or Legal Notices 84

Introduction

This book is not only about how you can live a healthier and longer life, but is also about how you can lose weight fast.

I will show you how you can use fasting as a way of not only reaching but maintaining your ideal weight and explain why for centuries it has been natural to fast. If you regularly fast, even if only for very short periods, you will be helping your body to restore its natural balance and use up the stored body fat currently sitting on your hips, thighs and other parts of your body.

There are chapters in this book that will explain what you should expect when you fast and what, if any side effects and symptoms fasting could have on your body. This is regardless of whether you do a quick 1-day fast or a full 7-day detox fast or even the hugely popular 5:2 Fast Diet or intermittent fast diet. I cover all of these and lots more in this comprehensive guide to fasting.

You may have recently heard that fasting is an ideal way to lose some excess weight very quickly and perhaps you need to do this for some big event or occasion.

This book will certainly help you achieve that goal but I also hope that by the time you have finished you will have a better understanding of what a fantastic effect fasting will have on your whole body and how it really can improve and lengthen your life.

I hope at the very least it will make you aware that it can be a way of keeping you as healthy as you can be, whatever your age. You will hopefully be pleasantly surprised at what other long term health benefits you will enjoy if you fast even 1 day a month.

I have put together some important information as well as a very short history of fasting that I hope you will find interesting and helpful and I do mean short.

So let's get going and try to get a lot healthier as well as lose some serious weight.

Is Fasting a Good Idea?

One of the first questions I asked when looking in to fasting as a quick way of losing weight was:-

Is Fasting a Good Idea?

Fasting is still widely associated with spiritual and religious practices. When we hear the word fasting we immediately think of Indian gurus or Buddhist holy men or even practicing Catholics who fast during Lent. Let's not forget the millions of Muslims who fast during Ramadan.

When people fast they believe that by doing so they will improve their clarity of thought and bring an inner peace. In fact many people today who do extreme fasts, say they achieve the feeling of being removed from the physical plane and are able to drift to what they perceive as a more spiritual consciousness.

It should be emphasized however, that practicing

fasting to this level requires you to have a strong and healthy mind. A good mental attitude is essential if you are going to make this work for you so if you are just looking to lose weight, the extreme fasts are not for you.

As you make your way through this guide, you will come to realize that you have actually found more good reasons to fast than you would have expected and hopefully this information will enable you to bring about the change that will enable you to extend your life.

If you have looked at other means of losing weight, you have probably read that to make any program work and more importantly be long lasting, you must complement it with a change in lifestyle that should include healthier eating. Fasting is really no different and it would be surprising if you don't change anything about your lifestyle once you know more.

However, as with all methods of losing weight, results will vary from person to person as we are all unique. Two people can fast under the same conditions but their outcomes can be quite different, so never compare your results with anyone else. What is important is that you when you begin to feel a positive change in your body you will change the way you think about food.

How Our Body Works

Our body is made up of cells, tissues, organs and numerous other systems that work hand in hand to keep us healthy and happy. They form a complex but harmonious relationship so that the absence of, or reduced capability of any one of them will greatly reduce the effective working of the body as a whole.

Our body has evolved into an almost perfect vehicle, a marvel of science in any age. The complexity of it and how it is able to perform so many things at the same time is still somewhat of a mystery. On its top form, it never runs out of battery although at stressful or overloaded times it will sometimes temporarily break down.

We have come to expect our body to do so many things. Each and every one of us are constantly testing and pushing our bodies to the limit and often beyond on a daily basis. I'm not only talking about physical exertion, there is also overloading it with a bad diet. We very often ignore the laws set by nature about caring for our body and then when our body starts to slow down or even fight back we wonder why.

Unfortunately most of us are not totally in tune with

our bodies. We are often unaware of what its limits are and sadly this lack of knowledge has led to persistent abuse over the years, especially when young.

We usually eat far too much at every meal and take for granted that the body will simply digest, absorb and then get rid of the waste caused by what we eat. We drink and smoke without thought and just trust that our body's defense system will sort it all out. Another thing we do is take common medicines on an almost daily basis and just trust that our body will cope.

Yet subconsciously we know that too much abuse is bad and our body is just like any other machine, once it reaches its limit, it will break down. This can happen if we over indulge in too much alcohol, unhealthy food and a lifestyle that lacks any form of exercise. Combine this with stress and the recipe is there for a gradual but inevitable breakdown.

As we age, our body will start on its downward path and carry on decreasing over time. As this happens, our body will become prone to different ailments and illness that we coped with when we were younger but notice that it is harder to do as we age. We will only become weaker over time and if we don't take notice of the warnings of our body, this abuse may cost us our lives prematurely.

We must always remember that our body should be handled with care just as we do with our other precious and irreplaceable things. We should always love and take care of it because transplants aside, we only get to have one.

What Makes a Lifestyle Unhealthy?

It goes without saying that a healthy lifestyle is better for you. We all realise that the cost of being sick in terms of time and inconvenience can be costly, especially if you work for yourself or have people that are dependent on you. So what makes a lifestyle unhealthy?

With our fast paced life, we are often lazy and depend on processed food and take-away meals more often than is good for us. We also as a matter of habit take many over the counter medicines and prescription drugs because they are widely available and easy to use.

We also tend to do less exercise as we get older than we did when we were younger because we tell ourselves that we are too busy to walk to our destination and usually end up taking the car or public transport instead because it is quicker and more convenient.

We are also exposed to many hidden toxins and chemicals in our everyday lives through the places we go and what we eat and drink.

Too much junk food is put into our hands especially into our children's hands from a very early age. We know that junk food often contains saturated fat which increases blood cholesterol levels and therefore increases the risk of heart disease and some cancers but we still find them convenient to eat.

Life is full of stress. Modern life is full of hassles, deadlines, frustrations, and demands. Work can be a very stressful place, whether in an office, a factory, or any other place of employment. For many people however, stress is so commonplace that it has become a way of life and they don't even realize how it is affecting them.

We have become dependent on medicines and are not aware that some have side effects that are dangerous to our health. Many people think that they need these medicines to manage their health problems but what they are not always aware of is that some of the drugs used to treat them can cause bigger problems.

Some of the common over the counter drugs, if taken too regularly are toxic to the liver and can do hidden things to your health and metabolism. Next time you are prescribed something or you buy a medicine from the chemist or pharmacist, read the label or the leaflet inside the pack very carefully to check what side effects may occur. Then decide if you need it or can do without it.

Exposure to pollution and toxic wastes such as hidden poisonous agents in many household cleaning products. Our bodies are absorbing the harmful chemicals present in the environment today. It is imperative therefore that we clean up our living space as much as possible. Those regular detergents, soaps, shampoos, toothpastes and perfumes that we use quite freely contain many chemicals which are toxic to our bodies, some even carcinogenic.

For a long time there has been a suspected link between breast cancer and deodorants containing aluminum. Switch to a natural crystal deodorant instead of using an antiperspirant. You can find these in most health shops and they really do negate odors without doing you any harm.

Lack of exercise. I could write a whole chapter on the benefits of exercise and how good it is for you and your body but you know that already. To put it simply, any exercise, no matter how small, always improves fitness levels and really does make us feel better about ourselves.

Fasting, What You Should Know

Fasting is often described by reference books as primarily the act of willingly abstaining from some or all food or drink for a set period of time. A fast may be total or partial depending on the reason for the fast and the period of fasting can be short, long or even intermittent.

Some fasting practices may even rule out sexual activity as well as food but this book won't deal with that type of extreme fast. Other fasts require you to refrain from eating certain types or groups of foods, for example from eating meat. A complete fast in its traditional definition is abstinence of all food and liquids other than filtered water.

We all know that over a period of time, the prolonged absence of food will eventually make us weak or have a detrimental effect on our body and eventually kill us. However, in controlled fasting this is not the case because water or other liquid is drunk in sufficient quantities to satisfy the thirst and more importantly to keep us hydrated.

The main benefit of controlled fasting is that during the absence of food, the body will systematically cleanse itself of everything except vital tissue in its search for nutrients. Starvation will only occur when the body is forced to use vital tissue to survive. Although protein is being used by the body during the fast, a person fasting even 40 days on water will not suffer a deficiency of protein, vitamins, minerals or fatty acids that can't be replaced.

During a fast, all essential elements are used and conserved in a most spectacular way during this breakdown of unhealthy cells. There is an unfounded fear in fasting that your strength will be diminished from the breakdown of proteins from your muscle fibers. This is untrue, because even during long fasts the number of muscle fibers remains the same. The healthy cells may be reduced in size and strength for a time, but they remain perfectly sound and will eventually recover.

A. J. Carlson, Professor of Physiology, University of Chicago, states that a healthy, well-nourished man can live from 50 to 75 days without food, provided he is not exposed to harsh elements or emotional stress. This is why it is useful to deal with the causes of stress before you do any type of extreme or prolonged fasting.

However, it would be one sided if I didn't say that fasting can also have a downside. Some people do excessive fasting out of fear of becoming overweight. Couple this fear with a history of mental weakness or excessive stress and you have the potential for a very dangerous and deadly illness known as Anorexia

Nervosa.

However, the fasting discussed in this book is for the good health and well being of the individual. Never use extreme fasting as a last resort to losing weight drastically. As with most other weight loss programs, good and lasting results only come with time and moderation. But that's not to say that it can't work very quickly, just don't use it constantly for quick fixes.

Other Uses and Facts About Fasting

Medical application.

If you have ever had to have a surgical procedure you will have been told to fast at least 8 hours prior to surgery. A surgeon or anesthetist asks his patient to fast because the presence of food in a person's system can cause complications during anesthesia.

Other certain medical tests, such as cholesterol testing (lipid panel) or certain blood glucose measurements, also require fasting for several hours so that a baseline can be established. In the case of cholesterol, the failure to fast for a full 12 hours (including vitamins) will guarantee an elevated triglyceride measurement. Patients about to get a CT scan are required to fast as well.

Political application.

Fasting is sometimes a tool used by political leaders and protesters to reinforce their protest, political statement or even to raise awareness for a cause. This is commonly known as a "hunger strike", a non violent method of resistance where protesters fast as an act of political protest or an attempt to bring about a change.

One of the most famous fasting events is that of Mahatma Gandhi who fasted until the violence in India due to the separation and partition of East & West Pakistan was brought to an end. This had a significant impact on the British Raj and the Indian population and ultimately brought about Independence for India.

In British history, one famous hunger strike resulted in the death of 10 prisoners in jail for political reasons. In Northern Ireland in 1981, an IRA political prisoner, Bobby Sands, was part of the 1981 Irish hunger strike, protesting for better rights in prison. Sands had just been elected to the British Parliament and died after 66 days of not eating. His funeral was attended by 100,000 people and the strike ended only after 9 other men died. In all, the ten men survived without food for 46 to 73 days taking only water and salt.

Fast Facts About Fasting

In an excerpt from the book "***Fasting to Freedom***", the author discusses the effects of fasting and how our body eliminates the toxins in the process. Here we are given an overview as to how fasting works and explains the positive effect and health benefits. These include an increased resistance to stress, increased insulin sensitivity, reduced morbidity and ultimately an expected increase in our life span

"During a fast, a metamorphosis occurs. The body undergoes a tearing down and rebuilding of damaged materials. There is a remarkable redistribution of nutrients in the fasting body. It hangs on to precious minerals and vitamins while breaking down old tissue, toxins and inferior materials. The end result is a thorough cleansing of the tube, membrane and cellular structures. This process of cleansing and rebuilding has made fasting famous for its ability to rejuvenate, heal disease and give the body a more youthful tone.

Eliminations during the cleansing process
- *Dead, dying or diseased cell*
- *Unwanted fatty tissue*
- *Trans-fatty acids*
- *Hardened coating of mucus on the intestinal wall*
- *Toxic waste matter in the lymphatic system and bloodstream*
- *Toxins in the spleen, liver and kidneys*

- *Mucus from the lungs and sinuses*
- *Embedded toxins in the cellular fibers and deeper organ tissues*
- *Deposits in the microscopic tubes responsible for nourishing brain cells*
- *Excess cholesterol.*

The Result

- *Mental clarity is improved*
- *Rapid, safe weight loss is achieved without flabbiness*
- *The nervous system is balanced*
- *Energy level is increased*
- *Organs are revitalized*
- *Cellular biochemistry is harmonized*
- *The skin becomes silky, soft and sensitive*
- *There is greater ease of movement*
- *Breathing becomes fuller, freer and deeper*
- *The digestive system is given a well-deserved rest.*

To heal illness, the body must pull all of its resources toward cleansing and repairing by removing appetite and reducing or stopping digestion. Wounded animals will fast, emerging to eat only after their wounds or broken bones have healed. This is the reason why there is little desire to eat food when sick, the body wants to focus all of its resources on cleansing."

Who Should NOT Fast?

Full-on fasting, no matter how carefully done can sometimes have a dangerous effect on certain people. It is strongly advised that these groups should not fast even if they want to. Here are the categories of people who should never fast or if they do, must practice extreme caution and be under strict medical supervision.

1. **Infants and children.** There is really no good reason for infants and children to fast. Due to their lack of maturity, they would likely not really understand the spiritual purpose of fasting, and their growing bodies need to take in ample nutrients regularly.

2. **Pregnant or nursing women.** Water only fasts should definitely be avoided by women who are pregnant or nursing. The baby requires so many nutrients for normal development and is dependent on the mother's proper nutrition to receive those nutrients. You are forcing the unborn baby to fast and can be potentially

dangerous to both mother and child.

3. **People with Cancer** - unless you are fasting in an attempt to help yourself heal in which case this should be under direct medical advice. Cancer is usually indicative of, amongst other things, an immune system that is not in good shape.

4. **People with other health concerns**. Water-only fasts should be avoided by those with significant health issues such as diabetes. However, juice fasts may be an option, but should be undertaken only under a doctor's close supervision.

5. **The elderly**. Water-only fasts should be avoided by elderly people. There is no need for the elderly to fast as their body may not be able to manage such a task.

And if anyone still has any concerns or questions, they should always ask their doctor. Remember, fasting is supposed to help bring out the best of health for us.

Fasting for Health

One of the most surprising but well documented effects of fasting is the healing process that the body begins during the fast. This healing process is said to happen as the body searches for alternative energy sources which you have deprived it of.

Because you are not using energy to convert and digest food, energy is diverted to another needy system, such as the immune system. This is why many people who are diagnosed with a life threatening illness are now investigating fasting as an alternative way to help with and support their recovery.

Properly carried out, fasting can promote healing, is rejuvenating and is thought to prolong your life. Fasting is actually all about the body healing itself if left to its own devices. This process is quite unlike conventional and alternative medicine which only deals with and treats the symptoms of the illness.

Ron Lagerquist in his book ***Fasting to Freedom***,

asserts that healing could be achieved through fasting.

He wrote: *"Fasting intensifies healing as deep tissue and tired organs are repaired rapidly. To heal illness the body must pull all of its resources toward cleansing and repairing by removing appetite and reducing or stopping digestion. Wounded animals will fast, emerging to eat only after their injury or broken bones have healed. There are testimonies of people's old wounds aching during a fast for the first time in years; unnecessary scar tissue is being broken down as fuel. This is the reason why there is little desire to eat food when sick, the body wants to focus all of its resources on healing.*

Why does fasting have such a powerful effect on healing the body? In the fasting state, the body scours for dead cells, damaged tissues, fatty deposits, tumors and abscesses, all of which are burned for fuel or expelled as waste. Diseased cells are dissolved in a systematic manner, leaving healthy tissue. The result is a thorough cleansing of the tubes, membranes and cellular structures. Ingestion of mucus-forming foods clogs the body's microscopic tubes and membranes, all of which are the highways used by the immune system. Fasting dissolves this internal mucus.

During a fast it is common for the nose, throat and ears to pass sticky mucus, clogging the sinuses. Strands of mucus may be found in the stool after the first bowel movement. There is a remarkable redistribution of nutrients in the fasting body. It hangs on to precious minerals and vitamins while catabolizing on old tissue, toxins and inferior materials."

Many experts in the fasting field, fitness experts, doctors and spiritual experts, would agree that fasting has a beneficial effect on the body and soul. Most interesting and informative is the article written by Gabrielle Lim, who summarized the benefits into five simple yet unforgettable sentences. In an excerpt from this article, she gives the 5 top benefits.

Retune your digestive system

Not many people know this but fasting can be a way for you to **give your digestive system a tune up.** *According to Dr. Naomi Neufeld, an endocrinologist at UCLA, "You re-tune the body, suppress insulin secretion, reduce the taste for sugar, so sugar becomes something you're less fond of taking." What happens is that the body eventually uses up the stored sugar (glycogen) so that less insulin is needed to help the body digest food. And that gives your pancreas a rest.*

Reduce your intake of free radicals

Mark Mattson, a scientist with the National Institute on Aging, has reported that fasting can **reduce your intake of free radicals,** *which can cause cancer. In fact, according to Mattson, "These free radicals will attack proteins, DNA, the nucleus of cells, the membranes of cells. They can damage all those different molecules in cells."*

Even just reducing your calorie intake can have the same effects as a fast. In a study amongst rats and mice, it was noted that those who were fed very little and restricted their food intake had a reduction in disease compared to those who were fed normal daily diets.

Speed up your journey to self-discovery

We are all creatures of habit and eating, just like smoking and sleeping, is a habit. What happens during a fast is that by taking away such an essential part of your daily routine, you **mess up your whole schedule**. This sounds bad but it's not, it's really a time to reflect on your routines and give yourself pause to think about how you want your life to move forward.

By fasting, you become more conscious of yourself and you can take the time usually spent eating, to meditate, write a journal, or do any other form of reflection.

Increase your gratitude

How could you not be grateful to break your fast? After each day when you do break fast, it's a celebration. It is a celebration for a completed day of fasting, reflection, and persistence. **So rejoice and celebrate your success!** Show gratitude to yourself and others.

When you break your fast, you will be very happy to taste food again. And contrary to some beliefs, you won't binge on food. In fact you will be more conscious of what you allow into your body and **feel gratitude for the food you receive.**

Launch yourself into your ideal life

Sounds like a pretty big benefit for something as simple as fasting, but it's true. When you begin your fast you can take this time to break old patterns, examine your current situation, and use it as the starting point for a whole new life."

Preparing to Fast

Depending on the planned length of your fast it can be helpful and almost essential to prepare yourself for the change to your eating habits and the mental challenges you are about to face. It would be foolish to read a bit about fasting and then decide when you wake up next day that you will fast. Plan your time, your activities and your mind.

Never go into fasting if you have an existing health condition without consulting your doctor first. If you are fasting to help alleviate this condition make sure you know of any problems you might trigger that could relate to your condition.

Now, if it's your first time to fast and you haven't done any fasting before, start by doing things on smaller scale. Try fasting for 2-3 hours or a half day. I know that doesn't sound a lot but if you find that really easy, step it up a notch. In no time you will have slipped into fasting without even realizing it. Don't forget, we fast for sometimes 7-8 hours every time we go to sleep. This is why the first meal of the day is called break-fast. We are only going to extend this natural way of resting our digestive and immune system.

When you decide that evening to fast the next day, try going to sleep without eating anything else. You can then try carrying on and fasting for the whole morning to see how you get on. Don't try the whole day fast or the 1 week fast straightaway as your body and your willpower could be overwhelmed, unless you really feel you could cope. Start slowly and build it up, get your mind and body used to going without food for short periods and it will soon accept the longer time when you are ready.

When you are preparing to do a long fast, try to eat one single meal a day for a few days prior to starting the main fast. Try to slowly cut-down your caffeine, alcohol or smoking habits for the preceding days. If you're a little bolder, try to eat nothing but fruits and vegetables for a set amount of time, and cut out meat products for that week. It shouldn't be too difficult as vegetarians manage it without going hungry. Whatever kind of trial fast you manage to do, it will give you a fair idea of what to expect when you commit to a more serious fast.

There is no doubt that fasting will be difficult for you if your diet contains large amounts of red meat, processed foods and/or if you drink a lot of tea and coffee or are a smoker. Sudden caffeine withdrawal can induce headaches if you are used to having caffeine throughout the day. Cutting back or altering your diet for a few days before you fast can help your body with the detoxification process and will then be less of a shock once you get into your fast.

Most would agree that fasting detoxifies the body. By eating less or nothing at all your body has an opportunity to cleanse itself in a way it wouldn't normally have the chance to do.

Here are some common sense steps to take when considering when to start any type of fast

- Determine how long you are initially going to fast for and stick to it.
- Plan to have a day of low activity or take some time off for the period of your fast.
- Avoid heavy work of any kind if at all possible.

The bottom line is that when you are ready to try a long fast, just do the best you can. Your body knows its job and when your fast causes it to increase its detoxification, the liver, kidneys, lungs and immune system will work extra hard to handle the load. This is why it is a good idea to prepare beforehand as mentioned above, as the purpose of preparation is so that your body will not be shocked and overwhelmed by it all.

Stages of Fasting

Below is an excerpt from the book "*How and When to Be Your Own Doctor*" book, by Dr. Isabelle A. Moser with Steve Solomon, published in 1997. It clearly described the various stages of fasting and how they work in relation to your body.

"The best way to understand what happens when we fast is to break up the process into six stages: preparation for the fast, loss of hunger, acidosis, normalization, healing, and breaking the fast.

A person that has consumed the typical Western diet most of their life and whose life is not in immediate danger would be very wise to gently prepare their body for the fast. Two weeks would be a minimum amount of time, and if the prospective faster wants an easier time of it, they should allow a month or even two for preliminary housecleaning During this time, eliminate all meat, fish, dairy products, eggs, coffee, black tea, salt, sugar, alcohol, drugs, cigarettes, and greasy foods. This de-addiction will make the process of fasting much more pleasant, and is strongly recommended.

However, eliminating all these harmful substances is withdrawal from addictive substances and will not be easy for most. I have more to say about this later when I talk about allergies and addictions.

The second stage, **psychological hunger**, *is usually felt as an intense desire for food. This passes within three or four days of not eating anything. Psychological hunger usually begins with the first missed meal. If the faster seems to be losing their resolve, I have them drink unlimited quantities of good-tasting herb teas, (sweetened --only if absolutely necessary, with NutraSweet). Salt-free* *broths made from meatless instant powder (obtainable at the health food store) can also fend off the desire to eat until this stage of hunger has passed.*

Acidosis, *the third stage, usually begins a couple of days after the last meal and lasts about one week. During acidosis the body vigorously throws off acid waste products. Most people starting a fast begin with an overly acid blood pH from the typical Western diet that contains a predominance of acid-forming foods. Switching over to burning fat for fuel triggers the release of even more acidic substances. Acidosis is usually accompanied by fatigue, blurred vision, and possible dizziness. The breath smells very bad, the tongue is coated with bad-tasting dryish mucus, and the urine may be concentrated and foul unless a good deal of water is taken daily. Two to three quarts a day is a reasonable amount.*

Most fasters feel much more comfortable by the end of the first seven to ten days, when they enter the **normalization phase**; *here the acidic blood chemistry is gradually corrected. This sets the stage for serious healing of body tissues and organs. Normalization may take one or two more weeks depending on how badly the body was out of balance. As the blood chemistry steadily approaches perfection, the faster usually feels an increasing sense of well-being, broken by short spells of discomfort that are usually healing crises or retracing.*

The next stage, **accelerated healing**, *can take one or many weeks more, again depending on how badly the body has been damaged. Healing proceeds rapidly after the blood chemistry has been stabilized, the person is usually in a state of profound rest and the maximum amount of vital force can be directed toward repair and regeneration of tissues. This is a miraculous time when tumors are metabolized as food for the body, when arthritic deposits* *dissolve, when scar tissues tend to disappear, when damaged organs regain lost function (if they can). Seriously ill people who never fast long enough to get into this stage (usually it takes about ten days to two weeks of water fasting to seriously begin healing) never find out what fasting can really do for them.*

Breaking the fast is equally or more important a stage than the fast itself. It is the most dangerous time in the entire fast. If you stop fasting prematurely, that is, before the body has completed detoxification and healing, expect the body to reject food when you try to make it eat, even if you introduce foods very gradually. The faster, the spiritual being running the body, may have become bored and want some action, but the faster's body hasn't finished. The body wants to continue healing."

Additional Fasting Tips

Here are some fasting tips shared by author Debopriya Bose that reinforce the advice I have tried to give you. I think it sometimes doesn't hurt to have your views agreed with by other practitioners and the more often you read the same advice, the more likely you are to actually believe it.

"For those who do not fast regularly or are doing it for the first time, it is better to adopt a moderate approach towards fasting and then graduate to stricter regimes. Start with a 1 day program. Then move on to programs for 2 days, 3 days and so on. In between the fasting days, one can have food consisting of raw fruits, vegetables, soups and juices. This is a good way of graduating to a 5 or 10 days fast.

A first timer could consider juice fasting than water fasting as juice fasting is easier than water fast. Also a juice fast provides most of the nutrients and calories that solid foods provide. Hence one would not miss solid food when on a juice fast.

One of the important fasting tips is to prepare the body slowly for the process. For beginners, it is helpful to start fasting with a little bit of food each day. Extend the fast to 12 to 14 hours in the evening (including sleep). Such a method could also be adopted for a couple of days before actually starting the fast. For greater benefits from fasting, one should stop the intake of alcohol, caffeine, red meat, sugar and poultry for a few days before going in for a fast. Also the intake of nutritional supplements should be limited. Natural is the way to go during fasting!

For the first 2 days one may feel irritated and experience headaches. However, from the 3rd day onwards, one's body adjusts better to the fasting program. To avoid such symptoms, one could take a meal that would comprise of water, juices, tea or snacks made from fresh fruits and vegetables, sometime around 3 pm.

As it is clear that even during fasting, all the nutritional requirements of the body are met; there is no reason to stop working out. In fact regular exercise will help expedite the cleansing process. However, beginners can go easy with their workouts in case they are used to heavy workouts. Yoga and meditation are great ways to complement the healing process during fasting.

One of the important tips for fasting is not to start binging on food once you are out of it. Since the body has already got accustomed to eating healthy and only as much as required, fasting is good opportunity to start off with healthy eating habits.

Those who are underweight or pregnant should not fast. People who have undergone a surgery or are suffering from anemia, *hyperglycemia, and chronic problems of heart, kidneys or lungs should avoid going on a fast. Nevertheless, if one is suffering from some health condition it is always better to consult a physician before starting a fast.*

Fasting is not a crash course for weight loss. Despite all the benefits, listen to your body. If one feels ill while fasting, call in the doctor. It is important to follow the fasting tips in order to reap the benefits of fasting that ensures overall well being of the body."

NOTES

Methods of Healthy Fasting

There are many methods of diets & fasting. Below is a list of the different types or categories that are most commonly practiced. Choose the one that is best for you, your lifestyle and your goals.

Fasts that include foods

Milk-Banana Diet

In this kind of fast, 3 cups of skimmed milk and 3 bananas are consumed each day. You can add honey and lemon juice and lemon juice in warm filtered water during the day. This should not be for more than 3-5 days as the calorie count is very low and you will put the weight back on quite quickly when you stop.

Fruit Diet

In this type of fast, you only take fruit and fruit juices. Again, in this fast, water and lemon juice in water can be taken but this fast must not exceed 6-7 days, otherwise the body will become deficient of essential enzymes and amino acids.

Fruit and Vegetable Diet

In this diet, lightly boiled or steamed vegetables can also be taken besides fruits. But the use of salt must be avoided. This fast should also not exceed more than 6-7 days at a time.

Traditional Fast

In this kind of fast, a light meal is taken only once a day. This meal may contain a little of salt, sugar and fat. But you should not take any other fruit, vegetables, tea, juices besides that meal. Ordinary water or lemon juice in warm water may be taken as usual but no other liquids such as tea or coffee.

Fasts that do not include food

Water Fast

This is the most extreme fast and you can fast from 1 to 40 days. Try to drink 2 litres of water or more per day. The ten day water fast has become a recommended and popular option. Ten days on water will cause the same weight loss as 30 days on juice. But water fasting is far more difficult, especially if you have a fast metabolism.

Water fasting cleanses the body aggressively removing the toxins very fast. Water fasting can be more beneficial than juice fasting in combating persistent forms of cancer. It would appear to cleanse the tissues more aggressively but does require strict mental preparation. The less pressure and responsibility you have during water fast the better. Think of it as a holiday away from the normal patterns of your life.

It is recommended that the week before your fast, you drink fresh juices and eat mostly raw fruits and vegetables to cleanse the body so that the detoxification that occurs during water fasting will be less aggressive. Water fasting should always include two of three days of juice fasting before and after the water fast. This alternating between juice and water fasting is the most effective method of achieving a full and thorough cleansing fast.

Complete Fast

This is almost identical with the water fast above except in a complete fast you drink only a glass of cool filtered water roughly every two hours. You should be aiming to drink 7 to 10 glasses of 8 fluid oz each day. Water is the most important liquid we take daily so don't stint on these amounts. You can then take a glass of warm water with some lemon juice in, between the cool water times. The main purpose of taking lemon juice in warm water is to prevent gas formation and to help the empty feeling.

So to recap you are mixing throughout the day plain filtered water and warm lemon filtered water. Drink as much as you choose but not less than 7 to 10 glasses of 8 fluid ounces each day. If additional energy is needed during this period, then a spoonful of honey may also be taken with the warm water and lemon juice. You can also have the water of a tender coconut in place of the lemon juice.

Juice fast

Juice fasting is safe and less aggressive than a water fast. It allows the body to cleanse itself of toxins while greatly improving conditions for health. One of the benefits is that your energy levels remain high because you are receiving enough nutrients from the juices, allowing you to carry out your normal activities.

A juice fast will take the strain from your digestive system and free up some of your energy to speed up body healing. However if healing is your aim, water fasting does much better in that regard. Also, juices can replace any of the usual nutrients that you might lack through your poor diet etc.

Juices are easy to drink if choose the ones you like and use very little digestive energy. This will allow the body to put more energy into healing and rejuvenation. Most juices are packed with vitamins, minerals, living enzymes, antioxidants, photochemical, yet are still low enough in calories to force the body to feed on its unhealthy waste. This will enable you to push yourself along the path towards vigorous physical health and clarity of mind.

If you have read this far and not skipped to the menus at the end, you should now know and understand a bit more about the benefits of fasting, however still keep in mind that it should always be done in a healthy way.

Do not fast because you think you have found the latest fad for losing weight quickly and easily. It should always be done with the understanding of what this can do for you and your whole outlook.

How to Fast Healthily?

Be accountable.
Whatever the consequences are, be accountable for your actions and fast for the right reasons. Likewise, be sensitive to the response or reaction of family and friends who you confide in about your plans to fast. It is likely that they might have seen something detrimental in the press or on television about the dangers of not eating and will only be showing concern for you and your wellbeing.

Prepare in advance
When you have come to the decision to fast, do not act on the spur of the moment, it will work much better if you have done your preparation beforehand.

Make sure you know what appointments or events are likely to happen before, during and after the fast. It is always safer to prepare in advance for the things you are likely to have to do during the fast such as work or child-minding etc.

This time of preparation is useful not only for the body, but for your spiritual and practical levels as well. If you don't skimp on the preparation time, your fast will most likely go more smoothly and be much more enjoyable and effective.

Understand the effects on your body

If you have managed to read some facts and figures on fasting you will know that your body goes through several distinct phases when you begin to fast. It is possible that during the first few hours, you will feel weak. You shouldn't be too alarmed by this as it is natural as your body begins to eliminate the toxins in your system.

There are a lot more things that will happen but again, don't be alarmed as they are normal and will disappear as soon as your fasting is over.

Break the fast properly

You will be putting your body through a period of intense detoxification. If you are planning a prolonged fast rather than just a 5:2 or weekend fast, you should have medical guidance that includes plans on how to deal with some potentially serious issues once your fast ends.

The body has adjusted to a different state and you must not severely shock it by eating and drinking things that will cause discomfort as well as physical problems.

Simple Fasting Program for Beginners

If you now feel you have absorbed enough information on the effects of fasting on your body to enable you to make an informed decision to fast, you can perhaps attempt this simple fasting regime using fruit juice.

Begin by clearing out any junk food from your home even if you intend to do even a short 2 or 3 day juice fast.

Having cookies and potato chips in your kitchen as you attempt to fast will require enormous will power to stop you from eating them. Best to get rid of them, don't make it hard for yourself. You can give them to a friend to store until you finish your juice fast. Or donate them to your local soup kitchen or food bank. It is likely when you have done a fast that you may finally realize they are not really good for you.

Purchase organic fruits and vegetables from your local farmers market or the health food store. Organic vegetables are now in plentiful supply in most areas. If you can only purchase non-organic produce, avoid buying grapes, apples, or peaches as these items are generally grown with heavy pesticide

If you can't find or afford organic produce you can make a detox bath for non-organic produce by filling a large bowl with filtered water and 2 teaspoons of Clorox bleach. Submerge the non-organic produce only in this bleach bath for 15 minutes. Rinse thoroughly and drain.

Juice fasting requires you to chop, cut and peel assorted vegetables and fruits before you juice them through a heavy duty juicer so that you are consuming the vitamins and minerals immediately.

There is a huge difference in the health benefits between canned or carton fruit juice and the freshly prepared juices so don't make the mistake of buying cans or cartons. However freshly prepared juices will progressively lose their benefit after juicing and should be drunk almost straightaway. Storing fresh juices in your refrigerator for 4 to 5 hours is acceptable but avoid doing so overnight.

Combining fruits and vegetables is generally okay but there are certain combinations that you may find hard to digest or are simply not to your taste. A classic rule of thumb is that apples of all types can be juiced with any other fruit and vegetable as apples will digest easily for most people. Melons are best eaten alone because they tend to digest very quickly.

You may experience indigestion if you juice with foods or liquids that take the body more time to digest. Usually common sense and personal taste preference will guide you, for example, juicing carrots, bananas and kale together will probably not give you a juice you will enjoy but hey, everyone is different.

Juicing basics:

Prepare only as much as you will need to consume at each setting or you can juice for 2 or 3 portions at most.

For example a good snacking juice is made from juicing 2 apples, 1 small carrot, one half of a small lemon and ½ teaspoon of fresh ginger root.

For an excellent breakfast juice, combine ½ large medjool date (for the date sugar), 1 medium banana, and liquid from a coconut (or to cheat, use "lite" coconut milk from a can, if diluted 1 part coconut milk to 3 parts filtered water).

You can add filtered water to thin to your preferred consistency or not.

Juicing for lunch or dinner drinks could include combinations of any favorite vegetable and then add apples to sweeten.

For example, juice 5 to 6 large leaves of curly kale or dinosaur kale, ½ cup parsley, 2 stalks of celery, 1 large carrot and ½ teaspoon of fresh ginger root or cayenne pepper.

Try 6 leaves of rainbow chard, 6 leaves of baby Bok choy, beets (the tops as well), and a very small bulb of garlic for a spicy dinner drink.

Drink at least 6 to 8 glasses of 8 fluid oz of filtered water to help you adjust to the cleansing effects of juice fasting. If you intend to juice fast for more than a day, add 1 tablespoon ground flax seeds to any drink and consume three times a day. This is to make certain you are moving your bowels in the absence of soluble and insoluble fiber (as is usually found in the skins and cellulose of vegetables.)

Do not be too ambitious while juice fasting. Do not starve yourself by consuming too few juice drinks, you will only be hungry and give up too soon. Prepare from scratch and consume at least 5 to 6 fresh juice drinks in any 24-hour period along with the 6 to 8 glasses of filtered water. The water will fill you up as well as flush toxins through.

If you find that after the first 6 hours of such a juice fast you experience changes in heart rate (very rapid or slower than normal), dizziness, headaches, or extreme physical fatigue, consider limiting your juicing to only that 6-hour time frame. For example, juice Friday morning until noon.

If you are really hungry and miserable, consider breaking the fast gently with steamed vegetables, vegetable soup, plain toast and unsweetened organic yogurt. **Do not break your juice fast with steak and fries or a pizza.**

Depending on your general health prior to juice fasting, it is common to experience headaches and several additional bowel movements as your body begins to cleanse itself of the toxins. Move slowly back to solid foods by introducing steamed vegetables, easy-to-digest proteins such as scrambled eggs, yogurt, or chicken soup. Treat your body as if you have had a serious illness and are slowly recovering.

Remember to break the juice fast slowly so that you are not overwhelming your digestive system. If you experience what is called a "healing crisis" and find the juice fast kicks off a flu or minor cold bring your juice fast slowly to a close, adding vegetable and chicken soups back into your diet slowly.

Take plenty of rest as needed and cut back on very strenuous exercise while juicing. Light exercise, especially walking is fine and highly recommended

Notes

Easy Fasting & Detox Programs

I have included a selection of easy to follow detox and diet plans that you should follow as closely as you can but don't over analyze it. A lot of the days are similar to each other but rather than just say refer to day ??? of detox plan ??? I have given the actual instruction for that day to save you scrolling back and forth.

One Day Diet

To ease you into a more rigorous fasting program, this one-day diet is an excellent start. It will give your digestive system a well earned rest and allow any stored toxins to be removed. The one-day diet allows you to eat just **one type of fruit or vegetable** for a whole day and will not shock your system but will have a beneficial effect on your health.

With this diet you eat small amounts of your chosen fruit or vegetable more frequently during the day instead of the usual 3 meals a day. Follow the same guidelines regarding rest and preparation, choosing a quiet stress free day if possible.

- You will need 1-1.5kg or 2-3lb of your chosen food from below.
- 2 litres or 3.5 pints filtered water or still mineral water if preferred.
- Herbal teas or fresh herbs to infuse if liked.

Choose only **ONE** of the following to eat for the day. Make sure they are organic because they don't contain pesticides.

Grapes
Apples
Pears
Papaya
Pineapple
Celery
Carrots
Cucumber

The day before eat a light evening meal, do not stuff yourself in anticipation of being hungry the next day, this never works and will even make you feel hungrier. A vegetable or bean soup or light stir-fry would be ideal preferably no meat or dairy.

Have a nice relaxing bath or shower and go to bed early and relax.

In the morning start off with a cup of hot water with half a lemon squeezed in it. This will give the liver a boost. Do some stretching exercises which will stimulate your lymphatic system. Dry rub your skin to get the circulation going.

For breakfast have a portion of your chosen food and make sure you drink plenty of filtered water at regular intervals during the day. This will also serve to make your stomach feel full and stop any hunger pangs.

Late morning/Lunch/Afternoon, prepare and eat a portion of your food and drink plenty of water. Try to do some exercise or take a brisk walk, cycle or a swim. Follow this with some of your chosen food and a herbal tea.

Evening, finish off your remaining chosen food, relax and perhaps watch some TV, have an Epsom salts bath if possible and then go to bed early in a completely relaxed state.

Next Few Days. Take it easy over the following few days and ease your digestive system back into a healthy diet. If you can, start the day as before with a cup of hot water and lemon juice and some simple exercises. Eat light foods.

The Weekend Detox Diet

This diet uses freshly made fruit and vegetable juices
As with all other detox/diets, you should prepare a few days beforehand by easing back on your usual eating regime.

2 days before cut down your meat and dairy intake and also salt, sweet foods, wheat, tea and coffee. Avoid cigarettes and alcohol as much as you can.

1 day before eat only a very light evening meal preferably consisting of vegetables only. Try a soup or salad but do not eat meat or fish. You can have fruit for dessert but don't overdo it. Later you should relax in a fragrant bath and go to bed early, perhaps just read to relax.

Day 1

In the morning start off with a cup of hot water with half a lemon squeezed in it. This will give the liver a boost. Do some stretching exercises which will stimulate your lymphatic system. Dry rub your skin to get the circulation going.

For breakfast have a glass of your chosen freshly made fruit juice for your breakfast and make sure you drink plenty of filtered water at regular intervals during the day. This will also serve to make your stomach feel full and stop any hunger pangs.

Late morning if you can, try to relax as much as you can. Eat a piece of fruit like an apple or pear or some grapes. You can drink a herbal tea if you like them or have a cup of hot water if you don't with a little honey in it. Go for a walk before lunch, this will take your mind off things but also keep your metabolism fired up.

Lunch Have a vegetable juice of your choice.
Try juicing 3 carrots, 30gm baby spinach, 115gm cooked beetroot and 2 celery sticks.
or
3 carrots, 1 apple and 1 orange.
or
Any combination of apples, grapes, watercress, red cabbage, fennel etc. Anything you like will be fine, just get the combination that suits you. Try adding some coriander leaves and lemon or lime juice to flavour it.

You can also have a large salad using cucumber, tomatoes, carrot and beetroot. A dressing of olive oil and lemon juice will flavour it.

Afternoon again, relax and do some gentle exercise such as Yoga, walking, cycling or perhaps swimming. Make sure you drink plenty of water now and throughout the day.

Teatime Have another vegetable juice from the combination above.

Evening After 6pm but by 8pm eat a light evening meal of lightly steamed vegetables with brown rice. You can flavour this by adding some fresh herbs and some lemon or lime juice. If this is not to your taste you could have a vegetable stir-fry or a large salad.

If possible have an Epsom salts bath for relaxation and go to bed early but drink plenty of water before you go to sleep.

Day 2

You may wake up feeling tired but this is normal after yesterday's regime.

Repeat the same process as you did for day 1 but choose different fruit and vegetable juices if possible. **However do not have an Epsom salts bath today**. Still drink plenty of water and do gentle exercise only.

Days following your detox.

As with the 1 day diet, take it easy over the following few days and ease your digestive system back into a healthy diet. If you can, start the day as before with a cup of hot water and lemon juice and some simple exercises. Eat light foods only for a few more days.

7- Day Detox Diet

2 days before follow the 1-day diet by cutting down your meat, dairy and salt intake. Also take in moderation sweet foods, wheat, tea and coffee and try to cut out cigarettes and alcohol.

1 day before eat only a small light evening meal of steamed or stir-fry vegetables only. If you don't want vegetables, try a soup or salad but do not eat meat or fish. You can have fruit for a dessert but only 1 piece. Have a relaxing fragrant bath and go to bed early and read your favourite book.

Day 1
You will need 1-1.5kg or 2-3lb of **One** of the following:
- Grapes - apples - pears - papaya - pineapple - celery - carrots - cucumber
- You will also need 2 litres or 3.5 pints filtered water or still mineral water if preferred.
- Herbal teas or fresh herbs to infuse if liked.

In the morning start off with a cup of hot water with half a lemon squeezed in it. This will give the liver a boost. Do some stretching exercises which will stimulate your lymphatic system. Dry rub your skin to get the circulation going.

For breakfast, have a portion of fruit or vegetable chosen from the list above.

Remember to drink plenty of filtered water at regular intervals during the day. This will also serve to make your stomach feel full and stop any hunger pangs.

Late morning/Lunch/Afternoon, prepare and eat a portion of your food and drink some more water. Try to do some exercise or take a brisk walk, cycle or a swim. Follow this with some of your chosen food and a herbal tea.

Evening, finish off your remaining chosen food, relax and perhaps watch some TV, have an Epsom salts bath if possible and then go to bed early in a completely relaxed state.

Days 2 & 3

In the morning start off with a cup of hot water with half a lemon squeezed in it. This will give the liver a boost. Do some stretching exercises which will stimulate your lymphatic system. Dry rub your skin to get the circulation going.

For breakfast, instead of having your fruit or vegetable as in day 1 you should have a glass of freshly made fruit juice diluted with filtered water. Be sure to drink plenty of filtered water at regular intervals during the day.

Late morning try to relax as much as you can. You may have a piece of fruit such as an apple or pear or some grapes.

You can drink a herbal tea if you like them or have a cup of hot water if you don't with a little honey in it.

Go for a walk before lunch, this will take your mind off things but also keep your metabolism fired up.

Lunch have a vegetable juice of your choice. Try juicing 3 carrots, 30gm baby spinach, 115gm cooked beetroot and 2 celery sticks.

or

3 carrots, 1 apple and 1 orange.

or

Any combination of apples, grapes, watercress, red cabbage, fennel etc.

Anything you like will be fine, just find the combination that suits you. Try adding some coriander leaves and lemon or lime juice to flavour it.

Have a large salad using cucumber, tomatoes, carrot, beetroot and fennel if liked. A dressing of olive oil and lemon juice will give additional flavour.

Afternoon again, relax and do some gentle exercise such as Yoga, walking, cycling or perhaps swimming. Make sure you drink plenty of water now and throughout the day.

Teatime have another vegetable juice of your choosing.

Evening after 6pm but by 8pm eat a light evening meal of lightly steamed vegetables with brown rice. You can flavour this by adding some fresh herbs and some lemon or lime juice. If this is not to your taste you could have a vegetable stir-fry or a large salad.

If possible have another relaxing bath but do not use Epsom salts in it. Go to bed early but drink plenty of water before you go to sleep.

Days 4 & 5

Morning, repeat as for days 2 & 3 but you can have a fruit salad made up of 3 different fruits topped with a spoonful of yoghurt.

Late morning, Eat an apple or a small amount of grapes. You can have a herbal tea if liked and try to go for a slow walk before lunch.

Lunch, try a large bowl of salad leaves with a handful of sunflower seeds and if liked a dressing of olive oil and lemon juice to pep it up.

Afternoon, you should rest after lunch, perhaps do some yoga or pilates or some other gentle exercise such as walking or swimming. The trick is to keep busy to stop you dwelling on any hunger pangs you are having.

You should have another hot drink such as a herbal tea or similar.

Repeat the same process as you did for day 1 but choose different fruit and vegetable juices if possible. However do not have an Epsom salts bath today. Still drink plenty of water and do gentle exercise only.

Teatime, have another vegetable juice of your choice or if tired of liquids you can try a good handful of pumpkin and sunflower seeds mixed. If you don't like seeds try some vegetable crudités (sticks) instead, like carrot and celery.

Evening, you can have <u>**one**</u> of the following:

- A jacket potato with steamed or stir-fried vegetables
- Steamed or stir-fried vegetables with either organic brown rice or buckwheat noodles and tofu
- A large mixed salad with tofu with a dressing of sunflower oil and lemon juice
- A baked potato and a large salad with a spoonful of hummus on top.

Days 6 & 7

Morning, repeat as for days 2 & 3 but you can have a bowl of dried fruit stewed with fresh root ginger.

Late morning, eat an apple or a small amount of grapes. Drink a herbal infusion and then go for a slow walk or do some gentle stretching and exercise before lunch.

Lunch, choose <u>one</u> of the following for your lunch today:

- A large salad with a spoonful of hummus
- Pea Guacamole with vegetables sticks and rice cakes
- Warm vegetable salad with a baked potato
- Date, orange and carrot salad

For dessert you can have a bowl of natural yogurt with a spoonful of organic honey

Teatime, Have a vegetable juice of your choice or try some vegetable crudités (sticks) instead, like carrot and celery.

Evening, for your evening meal tonight try one of the following:

Hearty Summer Salad

Serves 3

Ingredients:
- 1x 15 oz. can organic chickpeas (garbanzo beans)
- 1x 15 oz. can organic black-eyed peas
- 1x 15 oz. can organic artichoke hearts
- 2 large organic tomatoes
- ½ large organic onion
- 3 large fresh organic garlic cloves
- organic olive oil and organic balsamic vinegar
- A few pinches of dried organic parsley
- Fresh ground salt and pepper to taste

Method

Drain chickpeas and black-eyed peas, and put them into a large bowl. Chop artichoke hearts (into eighths if they're whole, or into quarters if they're already halved).

Chop tomatoes and dice the onion and place into the bowl with the artichokes. Crush garlic gloves with garlic press and add to the bowl also.

Whip olive oil and balsamic vinegar together in a smaller bowl, then pour over the pile of vegetables and beans. Add a few generous pinches of parsley, then salt and pepper to taste.

Stir all the ingredients thoroughly with a large spoon to distribute them evenly and coat them with vinaigrette.

Enjoy............

Before you go to bed have a 2nd Epsom salts bath and go to bed early

The day after detoxing

As with all of the detox diets, take it easy over the following few days and ease your digestive system back into a healthy diet. If you can, start the day as before with a cup of hot water and lemon juice and some simple exercises. Eat light foods.

The 5:2 Fast Diet

The brilliant thing with the 5:2 diet is that you only have to cook low calorie meals twice a week so you shouldn't get bored eating the same menus, especially if you have a few favorite meals that you can have a few times without feeling too deprived.

I continually tell myself on my two fasting days that it is only one day and tomorrow I can have a pasta or rice dish or that chocolate biscuit or ice cream cone for tea.

The following menus are foods that I regularly eat and have adapted from my usual food shopping.

Some of the combination menus below will total roughly 600 calories which is fine for men. However as I am only allowed 500 calories I prefer not to use any of my allowance for breakfast and am quite happy to wait until lunch so I am in credit. This allows me a few extra cups of tea or coffee during the day in which I can have a dash of milk instead of taking it black, much more enjoyable.

If you really can't go without, have half a small banana or one of the newish breakfast biscuits which are only about 55 calories

Have one midmorning with a cup of tea and it will keep you going until lunch. You could always have slightly less salad at lunch or vegetables at teatime. Be adaptable but don't be too rigid. **Remember, it is only for one day**

Breakfast Menus

Choose from the following easy to prepare Breakfasts

A typical fasting-day breakfast of 300 calories could be two scrambled eggs with a slice of ham (good sources of protein) or leave out the ham and you only use 140 calories

or

Porridge with Raisins and Honey = 224 calories, plenty of water, green tea or black coffee.

or

1 medium banana, 170g of 0% fat Greek yogurt, 1 tsp of chopped walnuts topped with a tsp of runny honey which is only 150 calories.

Breakfast 1 - Porridge with grapes

serves 1- 136 calories

- 30g Porridge Oats
- 200ml of water
- 50 gm grapes
- a dribble of honey

Method

In a large 3.5 pint jug or bowl, mix porridge oats with the water and microwave on high for 3 minutes, stir and microwave for a further minute, serve topped with halved grapes and honey.

Breakfast 2 - Scrambled Eggs with Tomato

serves 1 = 160 calories

- 2 medium eggs
- 1 medium tomato
- 1 tsp of fresh herbs for taste.

Method

Chop the tomato and microwave for about 45 seconds to heat. Do your scrambled eggs how you like them and just add the heated tomato at the end to serve.

Breakfast 3 - Toast

serves 1 = 140 calories

Method
Just toast a medium slice of whole-wheat bread and have a very thin coating of peanut butter. Try to get the no-added-sugar variety if possible otherwise have an even thinner scraping.

Breakfast 4 - Fruit & Yoghurt

serves 1 - 140 calories

- Half a small banana
- 1 pot Muller lite fat free yoghurt any fruit variety

Method
Just slice banana and add to yoghurt

Breakfast 5 - Fruit Platter

serves 1 - 100-120 calories

Choose 250 grams of your favorite fruit such as Pink or White Grapefruit, Pineapple, Raspberries, Peaches or Nectarines, Kiwi Fruit. <u>No Banana though.</u>

Method

Prepare and mix together your chosen fruits and then just weigh out 250 grams for breakfast on your fasting days. You can snack on the surplus on your other days if you like or save for your second day, will keep in fridge just fine

Lunch Menus

These lunches are filling but low calorie

Lunch 1 - Tuna Salad

serves 2 - 106 calories per serving

- 2 tomatoes
- 2 sticks celery
- 10 thick slices of cucumber,
- 2 spring onions
- Tin of tuna in spring water drained
- 1 tbsp of salad cream
- Good drizzle of Balsamic glaze

Method

Chop or slice all ingredients, mix tuna with salad cream and mix through salad.

You can use mayonnaise if preferred but add another 50 calories.

Lunch 2 - Poached eggs on Spinach

serves 1 - 120 calories

- 1 bag fresh spinach
- 2 eggs
- a little olive oil

Method

Poach the eggs as you like them. Rinse the Spinach and steam it for a couple of minutes by dropping it into a hot pan that has no extra added water. Stir until wilted and then drain off excess water by pressing into a sieve with a potato masher or other flat tool. Place on warmed plate and top with poached eggs and season to taste.

Lunch 3 - Mixed Salad with Avocado

serves 2 - 100 calories per portion

- 1 bag mixed salad leaves either rocket, watercress or any other you prefer
- 6 small tomatoes
- 1 ripe avocado
- Selection of fresh herbs such as basil, mint or chives (optional) olive oil and balsamic vinegar for drizzling

Method

Slice the tomatoes and shred the mixed salad. Mix with the herbs if using and divide between two bowls. Slice the avocado and lay on the salad and drizzle with the dressing.

Lunch 4

serves 1 – 109cals plus

Choose from the following
Kallo Organic Rice Cakes – 30 cals per cake
Ryvita Crackers for Cheese – 27 cals per cracker
Jacobs Choice Grain Cracker – 33 cals per cracker

100g Reduced Fat Cottage Cheese

Method

Just choose the biscuit you would like to put your cottage cheese on and calculate how many you can eat within your daily allowance. Top with a slice of cucumber or tomato, salt and pepper.

Dinner Menus

These are evening meals I have eaten often and are always enjoyable and low cost. If you prefer you can swap the lunch and dinner meals around to suit your busy lifestyle. Just stick within the 500 or 600 calorie range and you will lose weight.

Dinner 1
Fishcakes with Stir-fry Vegetables

serves 2 - 360 calories per serving

- 2 Fishcakes that do not exceed 300 calories per fishcake.
- 2 medium courgettes halved and sliced
- 1 tomato chopped
- 150gm broccoli cut into small florets
- 2 sticks celery halved and thickly sliced
- 1 vegetable OXO cube

Method

Cook fishcakes in oven as directed. In the meantime stir fry vegetables in a non stick pan, add a dash of balsamic vinegar and plenty of seasoning, a dash of water and crumble in the stock cube. Cook until just tender

Dinner 2
Vegetable & Bean Stew

serves 2 - 260 calories per serving

- 1 Onion
- 2 sticks celery
- 1 large Leek
- 400g tin Cannellini Beans
- 500ml vegetable stock
- 200g greens (either Spring greens, Sweetheart or Savoy cabbage)

Method

Chop the onion, celery and leek and cook in a little oil until softened. Add the stock and drained beans and cook for about 4 minutes.

Add the greens and cook for a further 5-8 minutes. If using Savoy Cabbage, cook until cabbage is as you like it perhaps a further 5-10 minutes according to taste. Sprinkle with a little lemon juice and serve.

Dinner 3
Chicken Parcels & Mixed Vegetables

serves 2 - 560 (280 per serving)

- 2 Chicken Breasts approx 125g each
- 1 medium onion sliced
- 2 small courgettes sliced
- 200gm green beans
- 1 medium tomato sliced
- 150 g broccoli florets
- 1 chicken stock cube

Method

Make 2 parcels using foil and divide the vegetables between them. Slice the chicken breast into 2 or 3 strips and lay on top of the vegetables. Make up the stock cube as directed and pour some into the chicken parcels, not too much, just enough to keep the parcels moist. Season well with salt and pepper and a tsp of your favorite dried herbs.

Fold up loosely and seal the parcels but make sure that you do not pack the parcels too tight or the heat will not penetrate and you will end up with undercooked vegetables.

Place in an oven proof dish and cook for about 60 minutes at 180c.

Dinner 4
Tuna Steak with Sweet Potato Mash

serves 2 - 325 calories per serving

- 2 Tuna steaks approx 100g
- 1 Sweet Potato - 400g peeled weight
- 2 medium tomatoes
- 150g of Broccoli florets

Method

Peel and boil sweet potato until soft, about 15 minutes, then mash with a little seasoning but no butter.

At the same time oven bake the Tuna for about 20 minutes turning over half way through.

Cut the tomatoes in half and place in another dish. Drizzle with a little olive oil and freshly ground pepper and bake for about the same time as the Tuna.

Steam or microwave the broccoli as liked.

Note: Sweet Potato is actually slightly higher in calories and carbs than white potatoes so you can have either. Personally I prefer the taste of the sweet potato but it's your choice.

Dinner 5
Mushroom Omelette with mixed salad

serves 2 - 680 calories (340 per serving)

- 150 g of mushrooms
- 4 medium free range eggs
- 150 bag mixed leaf salad
- 10 cherry or other small tomatoes
- Dribble of olive oil and balsamic vinegar dressing

Method

Slice or chop the mushrooms and cook in a non stick pan until soft but not shrunk too much, remove from pan and set aside.

Wipe out pan and spray with the 1 cal spray oil that you can get from most supermarkets. Beat the eggs together and add to pan.

Draw the eggs from the side into the middle of the pan until all of the egg liquid is almost cooked and no longer running.

Sprinkle the mushrooms on top evenly, season with salt and freshly ground pepper and when the bottom of the omelette is slightly browned, fold in half and leave to cook very gently for about 2 minutes.

Serve with the mixed salad, tomatoes and dressing.

Dinner 6
Tuna Steaks with Bean Salad

Serves 2 - 500 cals (250 per serving)

- 2 x 100g Tuna Steaks
- 150g mixed salad leaves or rocket
- 400g Cannellini Beans, drained & rinsed
- 2 or 3 garlic cloves, sliced
- Bunch spring onions, sliced
- 1 tsp olive oil
- 2 tbsp lemon juice

Method

Cook Tuna for a few minutes each side until cooked as you like it, or if using frozen cook according to packet instructions.

Saute the garlic in the olive oil for a few seconds and then add the beans and lemon juice. Cook for a few more minutes and spoon over the arranged salad leaves. Sprinkle over the spring onions and serve with the Tuna steaks.

Additional Meals

Try any of the low calorie ready meals in the chiller or freezer cabinets in most supermarkets. If you check out the Weight Watchers or similar low calorie meals you can usually find something to suit your taste for around 300-350 kcals that will fit in nicely with your calorie restrictions. If you are clever you can even split the low calorie meal you have cooked or bought between your lunch and dinner meal and achieve 3 meals a day. You really do have to decide what you can manage and it will be a case of trial and error.

Best Juicers

Just a short chapter about juicers. If you are seriously going to get into fasting whether it is full, part, intermittent or just want to be healthier, then at some point you will want to get a juicer. There are two or more types but the main ones are Centrifugal and Masticating.

Centrifugal juicers throw out the juice at high speed leaving the pulp behind. This action heats up the juice and kills some of the vitamin and minerals. If this does not overly worry you, then the cost of this type of juicer is a lot lower but they are harder to clean.

There are juicers that you are supposed to be able to put in whole fruits and vegetables and although this sounds time saving I have been told that this could put too much a strain on the motor and will not last as long

Even if you buy one of these I would advise at least cutting the produce in halves or quarters.

<u>Masticating Juicers</u> extract a more nutritious juice, breaking down fruit and vegetable fibres more thoroughly. However they tend to be more expensive but they will last a lifetime.

I have had my Oscar Vitalmax 900 for 12 years and have had no problems at all. Easy to clean and to use. You do have to take more time chopping up the produce but as you don't need to peel most things that really isn't a problem.

Conclusion

This has been quite a lot of information for you to take on board on how fasting can change your life as well as your shape. As we age we tend to listen to or read a mountain of information about improving our health and wellbeing because we usually abused our bodies when we were young and have only just woken up to that fact.

It seemed perfectly natural when the body was able to deal with abuse and heal itself quickly but as we get older the body system is not so robust and that is why we often feel sluggish and unwell.

However, during your research you will find there are still many doctors who warn against fasting for extended periods of time without medical supervision and who deny all of the beneficial points listed above.

They even say that fasting is detrimental to one's health and claim to have evidence to back up their statements. That is because they perceive fasting as just the simple deprivation of the body to what they consider much needed fuel. The idea of depriving the body of what society has come to view as so essential to our survival continues to be a topic of controversy. Bear in mind that some of these 'experts' will have vested interests.

There are a few myths and rumours on fasting, so much so that we don't know which are real and which are not any more. Having said all that, there are many reasons to consider giving fasting a try as a way of improving your health. The body is still an amazing thing as it carries on ridding itself of the toxins that have built up in our fat stores throughout the years. It also heals itself and can often repair some of the damage we have done to our organs during a fast. Finally there is sound evidence to show that regular fasting contributes to a longer life.

Let's not forget that the effectiveness of the fasting we do still depends on ourselves. How we view fasting and the reasons for the fast will still play a major role in determining our success.

All in all, the reason we fast may be about weight reduction, health improvement, or healing of the body. Regardless of the reason, fasting should not be scary and what's just as important is that we relax and enjoy ourselves as we fast. It should be a meaningful and beneficial experience for us, so just enjoy it.

Good Luck and all the very best of health always

About the Author

Best Selling author Liz Armond was born and educated in London, UK. She has been an active student of fitness and nutrition for over 30 years. She has always tried to lead a healthy lifestyle and looks for ways to get healthier and live longer. After trying out the 5.2 diet and having great success she put together her favorite recipes adapted for the 5:2 and published her complete series of cookbooks suitable for every diet.

Liz is now an enthusiastic advocate for this proven diet and is a firm believer that following this diet and maintaining a healthy lifestyle will achieve her goal of living a long and happy life.

She is married with two children and is an enthusiastic golfer, rambler. She also loves to ski whenever possible.

Other Books by Author

Recipes for the 5:2 Fast Diet

Vegetarian for the 5:2 Fast Diet

Vegetarian & Gluten Free for the 5:2 Fast Diet

Gluten Free for the 5:2 Fast Diet

5:2 Diet Meal Plans &Recipes

Vegetarian Meal Plans for the 5:2 Diet

Breakfasts for the 5:2 Fast Diet

5:2 Diet Meals for One Cookbook

Vegetarian Meals for One for the 5:2 Diet

plus

Fasting Your Way to Health

Mediation for Beginners

Disclaimer and/or Legal Notices

ALL RIGHTS RESERVED. No part of this publication may be reproduced or transmitted in any form whatsoever, electronic, or mechanical, including photocopying, recording, or by any informational storage or retrieval system without express written, dated and signed permission from the author.

DISCLAIMER AND/OR LEGAL NOTICES: Every effort has been made to accurately represent this book and its potential. Results vary with every individual, and your results may or may not be different from those depicted. No promises, guarantees or warranties, whether stated or implied, have been made that you will produce any specific result from this book. Your efforts are individual and unique, and may vary from those shown. Your success depends on your efforts, background and motivation.

The material in this publication is provided for educational and informational purposes only and is not intended as medical advice. The information contained in this book should not be used to diagnose or treat any illness, metabolic disorder, disease or health problem. Always consult your physician or health care provider before beginning any nutrition or exercise program. Use of the programs, advice, and information contained in this book is at the sole choice and risk of the reader.